Hypothyroidism Cure

The Most Effective, Permanent Solution to Finally Overcome Hypothyroidism for Life

Elizabeth Grace

Table of Contents

Introduction

Chapter 1 - Hypothyroidism

Chapter 2 - Possible Complications

Chapter 3 - Treatment Options

Chapter 4 - Natural Ways to Cure Hypothyroidism

Chapter 5 - Ways to Prevent Hypothyroidism

Chapter 6 - Permanent Solution for Hypothyroidism

Conclusion

Introduction

I want to thank you and congratulate you for purchasing the book, *"Hypothyroidism Cure: The Most Effective, Permanent Solution to Finally Overcome Hypothyroidism for Life."*

As the title suggests, this book contains useful information about a common thyroid disease known as hypothyroidism. We will tackle its causes, symptoms, treatment options and prevention strategies. Most importantly, we will get into the details of the most effective ways to overcome thyroid problems and provide a permanent solution to hypothyroidism.

Our society is constantly changing. Our hectic schedules and unhealthy habits take a toll on our health, though we sometimes do not realize it. The presence of processed foods and junk foods in our diet also has negative effects not only on our thyroid, but also on our general well-being. In this book, you will find out more about these and will be given a list of dos and don'ts towards achieving a healthier, more active physique.

Hypothyroidism is more common than you think. As its symptoms are often vague and tricky, some people with hypothyroidism do not even know they have it. This can be dangerous as it may lead to worse situations, if undiagnosed and left untreated for too long.

In treating hypothyroidism, you are not limited to just pills and other medications. There are various natural ways to restore your healthy thyroid and stabilize its function. Likewise, there are plenty of ways to prevent this disease and free yourself from the risks that accompany it. Staying healthy need not be difficult. Let this be your guidebook towards perpetual health and wellness!

Thanks again for purchasing this book, I hope you enjoy it!

This document is geared towards providing exact and reliable information in regards to the topic and issue covered. The publication is sold with the idea that the publisher is not required to render accounting, officially permitted, or otherwise, qualified services. If advice is necessary, legal or professional, a practiced individual in the profession should be ordered.

- From a Declaration of Principles which was accepted and approved equally by a Committee of the American Bar Association and a Committee of Publishers and Associations.

The information provided herein is stated to be truthful and consistent, in that any liability, in terms of inattention or otherwise, by any usage or abuse of any policies, processes, or directions contained within is the solitary and utter responsibility of the recipient reader. Under no circumstances will any legal responsibility or blame be held against the publisher for any reparation, damages, or monetary loss due to the information herein, either directly or indirectly.

Respective authors own all copyrights not held by the publisher.

The information herein is offered for informational purposes solely, and is universal as so. The presentation of the information is without contract or any type of guarantee assurance.

The trademarks that are used are without any consent, and the publication of the trademark is without permission or backing by the trademark owner. All trademarks and brands within this book are for clarifying purposes only and are the owned by the owners themselves, not affiliated with this document.

Chapter 1 - Hypothyroidism

Hypothyroidism, also called *low thyroid* or *underactive thyroid*, is a condition in which the thyroid gland produces abnormally low amounts of thyroid hormone. The thyroid is a butterfly-shaped gland located in the front of the neck, just below the Adam's apple. This gland is the master gland of energy and metabolism, and any complication with the gland affects many aspects of our health.

Since thyroid hormone is significantly involved in regulating metabolism - the process by which the body uses energy, people with hypothyroidism will have symptoms related to slow metabolism. Insufficient thyroid hormone also affects the body's normal growth and development, and influences various cellular processes. Depending on the cause, the thyroid gland may swell and form a goiter on the front lower part of the neck.

Hypothyroidism can be grouped into three main types: primary, central and congenital.

Primary hypothyroidism is due to the inadequate function of the thyroid gland itself, which results to a reduced amount of thyroid hormone.

Central hypothyroidism, also known as *secondary hypothyroidism*, occurs when some other organs interfere with the function of the thyroid gland, causing it to produce less than the normal amount of hormones. For instance, the hypothalamus and pituitary gland release hormones that stimulate the production of thyroid hormone. A disorder with either of these glands can cause an underactive thyroid. Hypothyroidism, which is due to a disorder of the hypothalamus is sometimes referred to as *tertiary hypothyroidism*.

Congenital hypothyroidism is the type, which is present at birth. Some infants are born with a thyroid gland that did not fully develop or does not function correctly. Some have an ectopic thyroid, which means that their thyroid is in the wrong position. Congenital hypothyroidism can result to growth failure and mental retardation if left untreated. To inhibit the development of these complications, most hospitals screen newborns at birth for any signs of hypothyroidism.

1.1. Causes

Hypothyroidism is a fairly common condition, which more likely affects older women. While it does not often cause symptoms or show any indication in the early stages, untreated hypothyroidism can result to various health conditions such as infertility, obesity, heart disease and joint pains. Several factors can cause hypothyroidism. These factors include:

Iodine Deficiency. Typically, primary hypothyroidism is caused by the lack of iodine intake. Iodine is essential for the thyroid to produce thyroid hormone and maintain its sufficient amount. Iodized table salt is a good source of iodine, so are other foods such as eggs, seaweed, dairy products, shellfish and saltwater fish. Contrariwise, too much intake of iodine can worsen hypothyroidism, so the right intake amount should be observed.

Autoimmune Disease. The body's immune system is responsible for protecting the body from infections and other invaders, but sometimes, the immune system mistakenly attacks and damages the thyroid gland cells, which then leads to thyroid gland failure. Scientists are still uncertain as to why this happens, but some think it may be due to a virus or bacterium, or otherwise caused by a genetic flaw. Anyhow, this process impairs the thyroid's proper functioning and lead to insufficient hormones. The common types of autoimmune disorders are atrophic thyroiditis and Hashimoto's thyroiditis.

Hashimoto's Thyroiditis. Also called *chronic lymphocytic thyroiditis*, Hashimoto's Thyroiditis is the most common cause of hypothyroidism. It is a type of autoimmune disorder characterized by the inflammation of the thyroid gland. Hashimoto's is associated with goiter (enlarged thyroid gland) and impairs the thyroid's ability to produce hormones.

Thyroid Surgery. Thyroid surgery may be necessary to treat certain conditions such as thyroid cancer, thyroid nodules, a large goiter, Grave's disease and hyperthyroidism. Depending on the condition to which the surgery is due, a part or the entire thyroid of the patient may be removed. If only a small portion is removed, the remainder of the thyroid may still produce normal amounts of hormones. On the other hand, removal of a large portion of or the entire thyroid can greatly trim down or cease the production of hormone. In such cases, the patient may need a lifetime supply of thyroid hormone.

Radiation Treatment. Radiation is used to treat cancers of the necks or head and certain diseases, such as lymphoma and Hodgkin's disease. Some patients with thyroid cancer, nodular goiter or Grave's disease undergo radioactive iodine treatment to destroy their thyroid gland purposely. These treatments damage the thyroid and can partially or completely lose its function.

Medications. Certain medications for cancer, psychiatric disorders and heart conditions can interfere with the production of thyroid hormone, leading to hypothyroidism. These medicines include lithium, amiodarone, interleukin-2, and interferon alpha.

Pituitary Gland Disorder. The pituitary gland produces TSH or thyroid-stimulating hormone, which signals the thyroid to make enough thyroid hormones. When a surgery, radiation or tumor cause's damage to the pituitary gland, the thyroid may no longer get the "signal" it needs from the pituitary gland, causing it to fail in producing enough hormone.

Pregnancy. Hypothyroidism occurs in some women during pregnancy. This is often due to the production of antibodies to the thyroid gland. If untreated, this condition may increase the risk of premature delivery or miscarriage. Some women may also develop a condition called *postpartum thyroiditis* after pregnancy. This condition causes them to have a massive increase in hormone production followed by a severe decline in thyroid hormone levels. This type of thyroiditis is usually transient and recovers in time.

1.2.   Symptoms

People with hypothyroidism usually display mild or no symptoms at all, depending on the severity and duration of the thyroid hormone deficiency. But generally, the common signs and symptoms of hypothyroidism include the following:

- Weight gain

- Hair loss

- Weakness

- Fatigue

- Reduced tolerance to cold

- Dry and coarse hair

- Irritability

- Muscle cramps and aches

- Impaired memory

- Rough and pale skin

- Constipation

- Irregular menstrual cycles

- Decreased or loss of libido

- Puffy face

- Hoarse voice

- Thinning hair

- Slow heart rate

- Poor hearing

- Decreased concentration

- Excessive sleepiness

- Loss of appetite

- Depression

Symptoms of hypothyroidism are often vague and can be attributed to aging or other conditions. However, if not treated, the signs can gradually worsen, leading to the development of more severe illnesses. If you have any of these symptoms, it is best to consult your doctor for proper diagnosis.

1.3. Diagnosis

The accurate diagnosis of hypothyroidism is based on the following:

Symptoms. Hypothyroidism does not have any distinctive symptoms. The symptoms listed above are not always evident in patients with hypothyroidism and can occur in people with different health conditions. Nevertheless, it will be helpful to disclose to your doctor any sign or symptom that you may have and for how long you have had them. This is a way to determine whether the symptoms are due to hypothyroidism or not.

Medical History. To diagnose hypothyroidism, the doctor will ask you if:

(a) you are experiencing any change in your health that may imply that your body is decelerating;

(b) you have undergone thyroid surgery;

(c) you have received radiation treatment to your neck or head;

(d) you are taking any medication that can lead to hypothyroidism (e.g. lithium, amiodarone, interleukin-2, or interferon alpha);

(e) anyone in your family or near relations has thyroid condition.

Blood Tests. Through blood tests, doctors can measure the levels of TSH (thyroid-stimulating hormone) and thyroid hormone thyroxine in the blood. If you have an underactive thyroid, the thyroxine level in your blood is low and the TSH level is high. This is because the pituitary gland releases more TSH in an attempt to trigger the thyroid gland to release more thyroid hormone.

TSH Test. The TSH test measures the amount of thyroid hormone thyroxine or T4 that your thyroid gland is being told to produce. If the TSH is abnormally high, it means that your thyroid is underactive. If the T4 in the blood is inadequate, the thyroid gland is told to produce more T4.

T4 Test. Doctors use this test to measure the actual amount of thyroid hormone circulating in the blood. Abnormally low level of T4 indicates hypothyroidism.

Physical Exam. Physical exam include checking your thyroid gland and looking for changes in the body such as swelling, slowed heart rate, impaired reflexes, dry skin and so on.

Chapter 2 - Possible Complications

If not treated immediately, the symptoms of hypothyroidism will progress and may eventually lead to other complications including:

Goiter

If the thyroid is constantly stimulated to produce more hormones due to inadequacy, it may swell and lead to goiter. This condition is commonly caused by Hashimoto's thyroiditis, a type of thyroid inflammation, which occurs when the patient's own immune system attacks the thyroid gland. A large goiter is not generally uncomfortable, but it can affect the patient's physical appearance and interfere with breathing or swallowing.

Infertility

Low thyroid hormone levels can get in the way of ovulation and may result to infertility. Additionally, autoimmune diseases and other causes of underactive thyroid can also result to infertility.

Birth Defects

A baby born to a woman with untreated thyroid disorder is more susceptible to birth defects than a baby born to a healthy mother. The baby may also have a higher risk of grave developmental and intellectual problems. Moreover, infants with congenital hypothyroidism are prone to serious complications with both mental and physical development if the condition is left untreated. For this reason, most newborns are screened for any signs of thyroid problems to eliminate any risk of future complications.

Heart Diseases

An underactive thyroid can also heighten the levels of LDL or low density lipoprotein in the blood. LDL is a bad type of cholesterol that can foster certain heart diseases. Even people with undeveloped symptoms of hypothyroidism can have an increased cholesterol levels and impaired heart functions. An underactive thyroid can also cause heart failure and enlarged heart.

Peripheral Neuropathy

The peripheral nerves are the nerves that relay messages to and from the brain. If untreated for too long, an underactive thyroid can cause impairment to these nerves and lead to peripheral neuropathy. People with this condition may feel pain, tingling and numbness in the areas served by the damaged nerve. Other symptoms may include reduced muscle control and muscle weakness.

Mental Health Concerns

Hypothyroidism can cause depression in some patients. It can also affect mental functions that may worsen as the thyroid disorder grows more severe.

Myxedema Coma

Extreme, undiagnosed hypothyroidism can lead to a rare, but life-threatening condition known as myxedema. This is the most severe and profound form of hypothyroidism in which the patient becomes unresponsive and loses consciousness. There are even cases when the patient suffers from a coma. The patient can also have low blood pressure, decreased body temperature and decreased breathing. In worst cases, myxedema coma can lead to death. If you have severe hypothyroidism or symptoms of myxedema, you will need immediate medical treatment.

Chapter 3 - Treatment Options

Hypothyroidism is totally treatable in most cases. The aim of the treatment is to satisfy the lack of thyroid hormone and bring the TSH and T4 levels back to normal. In treating hypothyroidism, the most commonly recommended medicine is a thyroid hormone pill called Levothyroxine.

Levothyroxine, a synthetic replacement for T4, restores sufficient hormone levels and reverses the symptoms of hypothyroidism. The dosage for this medicine varies for each patient, depending on the severity of the thyroid disorder. Initially, the doctor checks the TSH level of the patient to determine the appropriate dosage. The dosage is then re-evaluated and adjusted over the few succeeding months until the normal range is established. Your doctor is also likely to check the levels of your TSH every year and re-evaluate the dose as needed.

It is important to take the right dosage for Levothyroxine. Excessive hormone amounts can cause side effects such as insomnia, shakiness, palpitations and increased appetite. Levothyroxine is fairly inexpensive and, if taken in the right dose, does not come with any side effects. In case you need to switch brands, discuss it with your doctor to make sure you are still getting the appropriate dosage.

Besides Levothyroxine, there are other treatment options for hypothyroidism. These medications include Natural Desiccated Thyroid (NDT), Liothyronine, and Lactose-free Levothyroxine.

Natural Desiccated Thyroid

Before Levothyroxine (T4) came on the market, Natural Desiccated Thyroid or NDT tablets were given. NDT is an extract from animals' (usually pigs') thyroid glands and it contains forms of T4 and T3. It also has calcitonin, a type of hormone involved in regulating calcium levels.

Although it used to be known as an effective treatment for hypothyroidism, NDT is rarely prescribed by doctors today. American professional guidelines and British Thyroid Association also do not encourage its use.

Lactose-free Levothyroxine

For patients who are lactose intolerant or are intolerant of binders and fillers present in a levothyroxine tablet, Lactose-free

Levothyroxine may be recommended. These tablets do not contain certain ingredients, but still have the effect needed to treat hypothyroidism.

Liothyronine (T3)

Aside from thyroxine (T4), the thyroid gland makes another hormone called triiodothyronine (T3). T3 is the more active hormone and performs more quickly than T4.

People with hypothyroidism who achieve little or no improvement despite taking optimal dosage of levothyroxine (T4) may request adjunctive medication with Liothyronine (T3). Although this combination treatment still lacks evidence as to its efficacy, some people declare that they feel better when they receive treatment with the addition of T3. Since T3 is short-lived, it is crucial to take Liothyronine more frequently.

Most patients usually feel improvement within the first few weeks of taking medication and the symptoms typically disappear after a few months. However, you should not stop taking the medication once you feel better. Otherwise, the symptoms of hypothyroidism may return. You need to take the prescribed drug as directed by your doctor.

Chapter 4 - Natural Ways to Cure Hypothyroidism

While severe cases of hypothyroidism may require immediate medication, most mild to moderate cases can be cured naturally. Medications can be addictive and your body tends to be dependent on them. If you're already taking medication for hypothyroidism, you may gradually wean yourself from it. Sudden interruption of such medications will cause severe fatigue and may result to further thyroid complications. Always seek your doctor's advice first before altering your method of treatment.

As with any other medical condition, your diet and exercise habits greatly influence hypothyroidism. Eating the right foods and getting proper exercise is the key to curing thyroid disease naturally.

4.1.　Foods to Eat

Iodine. If you have hypothyroidism, you need to boost your intake of iodine (the other way goes for people with hyperthyroidism). Many table salt products on the market contain iodine so getting the daily iodine requirement should be fairly easy. Other sources of iodine include eggs, milks, yogurt, seafood and brownish sea vegetables like dulse, wakame and kelp.

Fish. Fish contains quality protein and are rich in Omega-3 fats. Insufficient fat can exacerbate hormonal imbalance, including thyroid hormone. Other natural sources of healthy fats are flax seeds, avocados, olive oil, nuts, nut butter and coconut milk goods.

Coconut Oil. Coconut oil boosts metabolism and encourages the thyroid gland to produce enough thyroid hormones. You can use coconut oil to cook with or take 1 teaspoon of this organic oil daily.

Fruits and Vegetables. Aim to eat local, organic foods like fresh fruits and vegetables. These foods are great sources of various vitamins and minerals that are instrumental in boosting your overall health.

Beans and Legumes. These foods are also good sources of protein. They contain many nutrients that help stabilize thyroid function.

Pearls and Apples. These fruits help promote hormonal balance, particularly in women. When mixed together, pears and apples create a powerful combination, which fights thyroid problems.

Glutathione. Glutathione is a potent antioxidant, which can improve the body's ability to regulate and modulate the immune system. Although glutathione is not present in many foods, foods like raw eggs, broccoli, asparagus, spinach, avocado, peaches, squash, garlic and grapefruit help boost the body's production of glutathione.

L-Arginine. Arginine stimulates the thyroid gland and thyroid hormones. It also enhances fertility and immune function.

L-Tyrosine. Tyrosine helps improve the thyroid gland's production of thyroid hormones. This natural amino acid also aids in coping with depression, which usually accompanies hypothyroidism.

Selenium and Zinc. Some studies show that severe deficiency of these minerals causes decreased levels of thyroid hormone. Foods like Brazil Nuts are rich in both selenium and zinc.

Water. Proper hydration is always important. It helps the body function properly and boosts overall health.

4.2.   Foods to Avoid

Soy. Soy interferes with the function of the thyroid and promotes hormonal imbalance. Too much soy intake can also increase the risk of goiters and other thyroid problems. If you cannot completely eliminate soy from your diet, try to at least minimize your intake of it.

Gluten. The thyroid tissue has a molecular composition similar to that of gluten. This means that if you eat gluten, you can increase your risk of autoimmune diseases like Hashimoto's disorder. Gluten can be found in foods made from rye, barley, wheat and other grains. Follow a gluten-free diet to prevent thyroid inflammation and regain the proper function of your thyroid.

Sugary Foods. As hypothyroidism greatly affects the body's metabolism, you can put on weight if you are not mindful of your diet. Eliminate or reduce your intake of sugar, as well as coffee and refined carbohydrates. Focus on non-starchy vegetables and foods that are high in nutrients.

Processed Foods. To help your body heal itself from hypothyroidism, refrain from eating foods that can burden your immune system. These include all processed foods, preservatives, color, white sugar, white flour, aluminum, hydrogenated oils, high-fructose corn syrup and other related products. Organic foods are the best way to go.

Red Meat. Resolve to eat less meat, especially red meat. If unavoidable, ensure that the beef is hormone-free and is grass-fed because this has a higher natural ratio of omega-6 and omega-3 fats.

Canola Oil. Canola oil inhibits thyroid hormone production, amongst its several hazards. Use only organic oil and consider canola oil a dreadful poison.

Alcohol. Alcohol intake can reduce your thyroid's ability to produce hormone and bring your thyroid hormone to abnormally low levels. Alcohol also has a toxic consequence on the thyroid gland and stifles the body's ability to use thyroid hormone. If you have hypothyroidism, completely eliminate alcohol or drink in cautious moderation.

4.3. Proper Exercise

To cure hypothyroidism naturally, find a physical activity, which you find enjoyable and do it regularly. Exercise promotes blood circulation and proper distribution of thyroid hormone to every cell. Curing hypothyroidism is not possible without the benefits of a good exercise.

Join a fitness class. To make it more encouraging, get yourself involved in group fitness activities. There are several approaches to health and wellness. You can join sports classes or participate in yoga, meditation or tai chi sessions. Exercise does not need to be vigorous. Even brisk walking for thirty minutes will do. Get an exercise buddy and strive to do physical activities on a daily basis.

Ease your stress. Identify the specific areas in your life that bring about stress and resolve to reduce their negative effects on you. Learn relaxation techniques, such as deep breathing, meditation or visualization.

Give yourself time to rest. Get enough sleep time at night and allow yourself to relax amidst your daily activities. The thyroid is one of the glands, which reacts to stress and can get too much affected by high stress levels. For this reason, you need to rest and relax to give your thyroid enough time to "reboot."

4.4. Other Recommendations

No BPA. Most plastic bottles contain BPA or Bisphenol A, which upsets the endocrine system and negatively affect the thyroid. Use glass or stainless steel when drinking to avoid the harmful effects of BPA.

Detox heavy metal. Use a combination of chlorella, turmeric, cilantro and milk thistle to eliminate toxic metals from your organs and cells.

Balance estrogen levels. For women, too much estrogen impedes thyroid function. To balance estrogen levels, eliminate birth control pills, increase fiber in your diet to a normal amount and avoid all non-organic foods. Also, cut down your dairy intake as milk usually contains high amounts of estrogen.

Stick to an alkaline diet. An alkaline diet can be greatly beneficial in treating chronic disorders including thyroid diseases.

Be mindful of your iodine levels. While it is recommended to increase your iodine intake if you have hypothyroidism, you still need to be wary lest your intake becomes excessive. Too much iodine can worsen your thyroid problem and lead to other health conditions.

Acknowledge adrenal fatigue. There is a close connection between the adrenal glands and thyroid. Patients with hypothyroidism usually experience adrenal fatigue as well. Do not ignore these signs. It can help identify early development of thyroid disorders and inhibit their building up early on.

Proper diet and exercise often goes hand in hand in treating any kind of medical condition. Knowing which foods trigger thyroid diseases and striving to avoid them can seriously help you cope with your condition. As proper exercise is beneficial various ways, take time to do regular physical activities and practice relaxation. This will improve not only your thyroid function, but also your overall health.

Endeavor to include these wellness tips into your daily routine while treating your hypothyroidism and even after your full recovery. Breaking out of your healthy lifestyle just because you feel better may encourage the return of previous thyroid disorders.

Chapter 5 - Ways to Prevent Hypothyroidism

As often said, prevention is better than cure. While there are really no conclusive ways to prevent hypothyroidism, there are ways to lower your risk of acquiring any kind of thyroid disorder. Here are some suggestions to help prevent hypothyroidism:

Resolve to quit smoking

Smoking really does not do anyone good. It adversely damages most of our vital organs and the consequences are often severe, so it shouldn't be any surprise that smoking has a negative impact on our thyroid as well. Aside from the numerous health problems associated with smoking, it can also increase your risk of thyroid diseases such as Grave's disease (an autoimmune disorder that often leads to hyperthyroidism), hyperthyroidism itself, and hypothyroidism.

Tobacco smoke contains many toxins that are particularly hazardous to the thyroid and can initiate thyroid disease in vulnerable people. One in particular is cyanide, which then converts into thiocyanate. This toxin directly inhibits hormone production and iodide (the ion state of iodine) uptake. It can be difficult to quit smoking but there are various support groups and other strategies that you can try— most of which have worked for many people.

Avoid all sources of fluoride

We all know that fluoride is good for our teeth; however, it can be bad for our thyroid. Studies show that iodine deficiency that may be due to extra absorption of fluoride is associated with hypothyroidism. There is indeed a tremendous increase in thyroid disorders related with fluoridated water and this indicates that fluoride has a restraining effect on the function of the thyroid gland. This further suggests that fluoride is the chief cause of hypothyroidism.

For this reason, some professionals recommend avoiding fluoridated water. Instead, drink only spring or bottled water, which is certified as fluoride-free. Also, avoid fluoridated toothpaste and treatments and other products that contain fluoride. However, some drinks like tea and coffee naturally have fluoride. In such cases, compensate the possible ingestion of fluoride by taking additional iodine.

Request for a thyroid collar when getting x-rays

Often when we get x-rays, the x-ray technician does not use a lead collar to protect our thyroid, thereby exposing our thyroid to excessive radiation. The thyroid is especially sensitive to radiation and unwarranted exposure to radiation increases the risk of several thyroid complications. When you need to get x-rays, either for your teeth, neck, head, or collarbone, request for a thyroid collar for added protection. The x-ray technician will simply place the collar around your neck prior to taking the x-ray.

Test for thyroid antibodies

Thyroid disease can be acquired genetically. If you have history of any kind of thyroid condition in the family, it is best to test for thyroid antibodies. These antibodies, as previously discussed, are predominant in Hashimoto's disease in which the immune system attacks its own body.

To get rid of thyroid antibodies, you may also take foods that can naturally reduce inflammation and supplement with selenium. Selenium improves thyroid conversion and consequently reduces antibodies. This in turn helps prevent certain kinds of thyroid problems and preserve the function of your thyroid.

Screen for celiac disease

Celiac disease is a condition characterized by your intestines' hypersensitivity to gluten. This causes difficulty in digesting food and absorbing essential nutrients. Symptoms of celiac disease include chronic abdominal pain and bloating, intestinal difficulties, gas, anemia, nausea, constipation, diarrhea, numbness and tingling in the legs, sores in the mouth, painful rashes on knees, elbows and buttocks, among others.

If you have any of these symptoms, get screened for celiac disease for proper treatment. You can prevent some cases of autoimmune diseases through early diagnosis and treatment of celiac disease.

Detoxify your home

Thyroid hormone disruptors are everywhere – in plastic bottles, cookware, pop cans, chemical-laden cosmetics, and many other toxic products. By getting rid of these things in your home, you can simultaneously improve your health.

A link between thyroid hormone levels and phthalates (common chemicals used in plastic) has been confirmed in various scientific studies. Exposure to these chemicals alters the function of the thyroid gland and causes it to make inadequate thyroid hormone - an event that eventually leads to hypothyroidism.

To further reduce your risk of thyroid diseases, get rid of the plastic containers in your home, especially in your kitchen. Always choose glass, wood or metal to store and serve foods. Avoid plastic as much as possible and use paper wraps that don't contain harmful chemicals (check with the manufacturer if unsure). Eliminate all toxic kitchenware and cleaning products to promote a healthier, non-toxic household environment.

Hypothyroidism can be such a nuisance, but when armed with proper knowledge of prevention strategies, hypothyroidism can be something you will never have to deal with.

Chapter 6 - Permanent Solution for Hypothyroidism

For most cases of primary hypothyroidism, the main cause is iodine deficiency in diet. Fortunately, this is fairly easy to remedy. You simply have to increase your iodine intake, make sure that you meet the required daily intake, and follow the other guidelines outlined in this book. Incorporate these habits into your daily routine and it will not even feel like you're medicating at all, but rather, you're just moving on with your life with a better perspective.

Although some cases require patients to take natural or synthetic thyroid hormone on a permanent basis, there are cases wherein patients can bring back their thyroid functions to normal by means of natural approaches. There are, in fact, some reports demonstrating how patients with viral thyroiditis regain their normal thyroid function after a series of medication. The same thing happens to some women after pregnancy. However, for most cases of secondary and severe hypothyroidism, patients will most likely have to make a lifelong commitment to medication. Hypothyroidism may not be totally curable in these cases, but you can completely control it throughout your life.

The real permanent solution to overcome hypothyroidism is to have the right mindset and self-discipline. Work well with your doctor to maintain the right dosage for your medication and take the medication exactly as you are prescribed. Do not skip doses, change brands or stop taking the medicine without the knowledge of your doctor; otherwise, you may not receive the appropriate dosage and prolong your recovery process.

Or better yet, prevent hypothyroidism before it even develops. Many thyroid conditions can be barred by maintaining a healthy, balanced diet, getting regular exercise, avoiding exposure to, and ingestion of, certain types of minerals and chemicals, and eliminating harmful products in your home. It is also almost essential to test yourself for various diseases and irregularities in the systemic functions of your body.

This way, any complication can be diagnosed and stopped before they even fester. By becoming more aware of your body and the world around you, you can create a sturdy fortification between you and any kind of thyroid diseases.

Conclusion

Thank you again for purchasing this book!

I hope this book was able to provide you with comprehensive details on how hypothyroidism develops and how it can be treated and possibly prevented. While some diseases are unavoidable, maintaining a healthy body and abstaining from bad habits can prevent you from developing any form of medical condition.

The thyroid may be but a small organ, but its function is big. It produces hormones that stabilize the rate through which the body uses food, water, fat and carbohydrates to make energy. It also helps control body temperature and normalize the production of proteins. Any alteration to the function of the thyroid can have adverse effects on your health, so it is relatively important to take good care of your thyroid.

There are various treatments for any sort of health problems, including thyroid problems, and choosing the right treatment method can be quite confusing. Before taking any medicines or alternative remedies, equip yourself with the knowledge of the disease and get advice from experts. Abruptly starting medication without proper diagnosis can lead to worse conditions.

Now, the next step is to change certain aspects of your lifestyle to make up for what's missing. Cut out the bad practices and replace them with healthier, more favorable ones. Hypothyroidism can alter your life in some way, but it shouldn't hinder you from having a fun and normal life.

I hope this book has given you some ideas on how to do just that. Have an enjoyable life and stay healthy!

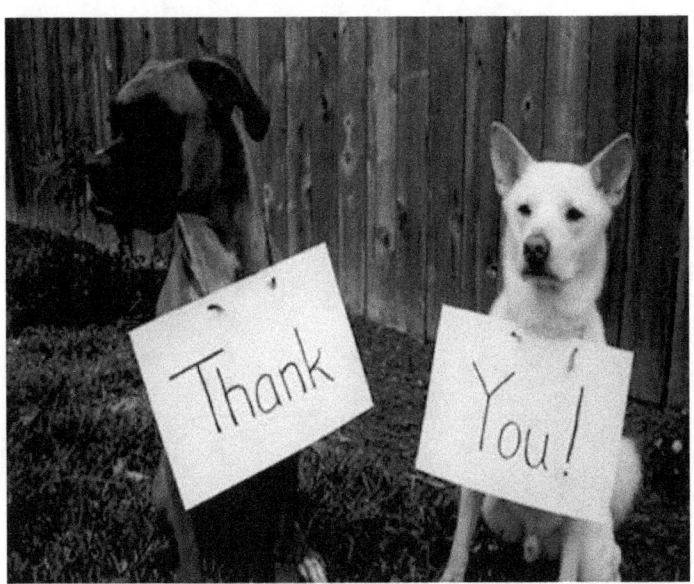

Finally, if you enjoyed this book, then I'd like to ask you for a favor, would you be kind enough to leave a review for this book on Amazon? It'd be greatly appreciated!

Thank you and good luck!

www.ingramcontent.com/pod-product-compliance
Lightning Source LLC
Chambersburg PA
CBHW070420190526
45169CB00003B/1345

* 9 7 8 1 5 3 4 9 5 4 4 2 7 *